A Routine For Healthy, Happy and Affordable Living

...during Times of Conservation and Global Warming

A Little Book by:

Paeti Gustav Xaviers

**THiS BOOK iS Dedicated to
ALL PeopLe,
WitH Love and Adoration**

**All products recommended in this book
should be available at**

WaLMart

Beauty Advice For the Young At Heart or Young In Age

Beauty for All Seasons

The truth about having a beautiful appearance that is consistent with your unique, personal self is to primarily follow the basics of living a respectful life, regardless of what may happen by chance or circumstance. There are certain quick things that anyone can remember to help guide them toward the ultimately serene appearance that may be longed for:

Follow Rules-

Rules are general guidelines that are already established and in existence for a reason. For example, the Golden Rule: "Do unto others as you would have them do unto you."

Other Basics toward Serenity:

"Follow your Heart."

"Do all the right things for all

the right reasons."

"Do whatever you legally want to do and try very hard to never hurt any other living thing, no matter what happens."

"Think before you take action. Think anything at all that you please, just do not ACT upon it before putting on your thinking cap and testing your idea for possible negative repercussions before actually DOING anything."

"Never Give Up on Finding True

Love and Happiness!"

Have a good, documentable reason when you feel your actions might be in violation of any Golden Rule. To Document your reason and help you think it out, write your reasoning down. This can be in a diary, a personal journal, a handwritten, personal letter to a friend or you can always depend on the Protective Arms of our United States Government (if you think your breach may have been a little against the law). If what you feel requires more than 3 to 5 typewritten pages, you can always start to write a book. For kids, the best bet would be to use a coloring book, creating a picture or playing with doll(s) until you can come up with a unique piece of colorful artwork that expresses how you feel.

ALWayS BeLieVe:

Always believe in the possibilities of your own self and never give up on achieving the image that expresses your natural inner beauty. If you don't FEEL beautiful at any certain time, but

want to express it, take a shower
first. Not a long shower. It can be
a quickie. This helps you wash
away all of the dead skin cells
that could be blocking the
absorbsion of necessary vitamins,
like vitamin D from the sun.

To encourage the natural
exfoliation of dead skin, wash
your hair, too. Be sure to
stimulate the scalp and use
shampoo scents that remind you
of something beautiful. Kids:
Take a bubble bath with your
favorite toys and play while the
warm water soothes your spirit.

And don't forget to say your prayers, every night if possible, before bedtime. That is, if it is not against your religion or the traditional beliefs of your family. If you cannot say prayers, cuddle-up under a comforter and get cozy. Magic can sometimes happen as quickly as overnight.

To get your share of the minimal minerals necessary to stimulate natural beauty, drink at least a glass of tap or faucet filtered water before bedtime. 8 ounces is fine. Keep thinking about what happened or what your desired result is until you can physically express your beautiful image in your own unique way. If all natural remedies fail, use a little make-up or buy some new clothes. Be patient. The natural healing that must take place as a result of just living takes time, depending on how hurt you may be feeling or how strewn your physique.

Keep Your Feet oN the GrouNd:

Mother Earth is called "Mother" for a reason. Take a walk, wearing the most comforting shoes and socks in order to thoroughly cushion your soles. You can even go barefoot for the fastest healing , but that depends on your physical location. If at the beach, play in the water. The natural salts of the ocean are absorbed by the skin and very good for you. You may just have to take a shower at the end of the day to prevent an overdose (sun and salt).

Kids, try swinging on the swings in the park while your voice reaches the tree tops. Try pointing your right big toe to the absolute top of the nearest tree in bloom and take focus with your right eye. Then smile. Sing to your heart's content. Sing your favorite songs or songs that you feel you sing well and have learned in school. You can also sing your favorite "top 10" tunes that you may have heard on the radio. You'll be amazed how many people will start singing with you to encourage you and help you feel better while feeling better themselves.

Always be sure to dress comfortably for the weather.

Don't let yourself get too cold. You'll shiver your spine, This could hurt the delicate communication nerves that are intended to help you heal in every way imaginable within the natural system, until you achieve your most unique, naturally beautiful self.

If you get too warm from clothing, start removing layers. Keep in mind, though, what is considered decent exposure. Indecent exposure is a break of the law, not just a rule, so be careful. You do not want to offend other people or things by your nakedness, regardless of how YOU may feel.

Still warm? Shower again in luke-warm water or wash you hands in cool water. Use soap. If your hands are overly dry or wrinkling, instead of washing, use a moisturizer and forget the water and soap. When you shower use soap scents that make you feel fresh and clean. Then be sure to put on fresh undergarments that encourage the expulsion of chemicals or substances that may be waiting to be replaced by newly recycled skin, tissue or whatever your body is trying to mend. This could result in a zit or cyst, but don't puncture those without speaking to a medical professional first if the size of it causes you concern or too much pain. The best colour for undergarments is white, which is a combination of all of the colors of the rainbow wrapped up in one. White undies makes a rainbow connection with your spiritual spine. Your natural beauty will become more and more visible in the mirror as time marches on. You will be amazed.

The Ten Commandments
Deut. 5.1-211

And God spake all these words, saying,

2 ¶ I am the LORD thy God, which have brought thee out of the land of Egypt, out of the house of bondage.

3 ¶ Thou shalt have no other gods before me.

4 ¶ Thou shalt not make unto

thee any graven image, or any likeness of any thing that isin heaven above, or that is in the earth beneath, or that is in the water under the earth:

5 thou shalt not bow down thyself to them, nor serve them: Ex. 34.17 · Lev. 19.4 ; 26.1 · Deut. 4.15-18 ;27.15 for I the LORD thy God am a jealous God, visiting the iniquity of the fathers upon the children unto the third and fourth generation of them that hate me;

6 and showing mercy unto

thousands of them that love me, and keep my commandments.Ex. 34.6, 7 · Num. 14.18 · Deut. 7.9, 10

7 ¶ Thou shalt not take the name of the LORD thy God in vain: Lev. 19.12 for the LORD will not hold him guiltless that taketh his name in vain.

8 ¶ Remember the sabbath day, to keep it holy. Ex. 16.23-30 ; 31.12-14

9 Six days shalt thou labor, and do all thy work:

10 but the seventh day is the sabbath of the LORD thy God: in it thou shalt not do any work, Ex. 23.12 ; 31.15 ; 34.21 ; 35.2 · Lev. 23.3 thou, nor thy son, nor thy daughter, thy manservant, nor thy maidservant, nor thy cattle, nor thy stranger that is within thy gates:

11 for in six days the LORD made heaven and earth, the sea, and all that in them is, and rested the seventh day: wherefore the LORD blessed the sabbath day, and hallowed it.Gen. 2.1-3 · Ex. 31.17

12 ¶ Honor thy father and thy mother: Deut. 27.16 · Mt. 15.4 ; 19.19 · Mk. 7.10 ; 10.19 · Lk. 18.20 · Eph. 6.2 that thy days may be long upon the land which the LORD thy God giveth thee. Eph. 6.3

13 ¶ Thou shalt not kill. Gen. 9.6 · Lev. 24.17 · Mt. 5.21 ; 19.18 · Mk. 10.19 · Lk. 18.20 · Rom. 13.9 · Jas. 2.11

14 ¶ Thou shalt not commit adultery. Lev. 20.10 · Mt. 5.27 ; 19.18 · Mk. 10.19 · Lk. 18.20 ·

Rom. 13.9 · Jas. 2.11

15 ¶ Thou shalt not steal. Lev.
19.11 · Mt. 19.18 · Mk. 10.19 ·
Lk. 18.20 · Rom. 13.9

16 ¶ Thou shalt not bear false
witness against thy neighbor. Ex.
23.1 · Mt. 19.18 · Mk. 10.19 · Lk.
18.20

17 ¶ Thou shalt not covet Rom.
7.7 ; 13.9 thy neighbor's house,
thou shalt not covet thy
neighbor's wife, nor his
manservant, nor his maidservant,
nor his ox, nor his ass, nor any

thing that is thy neighbor's.

THe DreaMS & NigHtMares oF HuMaN CoNScioUSNeSS

The Fascination of Dreams and Nightmares:

Dreams and nightmares are aspects of human consciousness that have fascinated humankind for ages. Since the times of ancient Egypt, interpreting the meaning of dreams and nightmares has been attempted. Some modern psychologists still devote substantial portions of their professional practice to the

dream and nightmare deciphering
attempt.

**So What are dreams &
nightmares and is there a
difference between the two?**

It has previously been discerned
by medicine that the human
being only uses a very small
percentage of their brain.
Meanwhile, the MIND consumes
the ENTIRE BRAIN. In fact,
dreams are a means by which an
individual is guided by the God
of their worship toward an
ultimate end, or destiny. If one

reaches an ULTIMATE END destiny, then perhaps they have chosen the incorrect God of worship (at least the last time they worshiped - or whom they ritualistically worship). A nightmare is like a "video stream" that God has the power to "imaginize" on your tongue, which is visible when daily consciousness is temporarily abandoned. Consider dreams and nightmares as lessons in "God School." How one responds or reacts to the dream or nightmare is FREEDOM OF CHOICE.

The Best Way to Get a Good Night's Rest:

If you experience dreams and/or nightmares that either frighten you or you cannot figure out what they may mean, separate yourself from inanimate objects that may be blocking the communication between your heavenly spirit (spine) and the soles of your feet (the door to your soul).

Do not sleep with earrings, dentures (or any other artificial object in your mouth). Your teeth take over the as communication projectors that create seemingly visual images. Wear a pair of white, comfortable socks (to the ankle is fine). Lie first on your right side, cuddle up to your pillow and try to fall asleep. If you still cannot fall asleep, carefully and gently, with your eyes closed, switch to your left side and repeat cuddle-up. If you still cannot sleep after trying to hold these positions as long as possible, continue gently switching sides with your eyes closed.

If you find it to be just impossible to sleep, at least try to rest peacefully on your right side until morning. Remember that God is Real, so you can always take a break. God is not a slave master. As God reads your mind when you get off your feet, His effort to soothe your life's miseries, one is always welcome to reconnect with Mother Earth by placing their feet back on the ground. Between God and Mother Earth you will find peace, eventually, as Nature's delicate balance is masterfully controlled. God considers

everyone's abilities, beliefs and
actions, and is very respectful of
an individual's feelings. Continue
this routine and eventually
nightmares will magically
disappear and dreams may start
to come true.

Dreams and/or nightmares are
simply the "videos" that are
created and reflected on the
tongue that result from the battle
that takes place between your
spirit's quest for physical, eternal
life and the actions you have
performed. One must effort to be
in control of their physical selves

as often as possible and
especially not to break a
religiously natural, physical or
LEGAL law.

Water: The Life Elixir

The Benefits of Water are Many.
Before you spend your hard
earned money on health and
beauty treatments to aid a
continuously aging body, do not
overlook the elemental ingredient
to good health and natural
beauty: Water. Think of this
"Adam's Ale" as a magical elixir
that can drive your physical self
toward an eternal youth.

* Water Helps Body Fluid
Maintenance

* Water Helps Control Calories

* Water Energizes Muscles

* Water Improves the
Appearance of Your Skin

* Water Helps Your Kidneys and
Maintenance of Normal Bowel
Function

* Water Intake Shines Healthier
Hair

* Water Naturally Thins Your
Blood for Improved Blood Flow
and Nourishment for Cells

Body Fluid Maintenance: It is probably no secret to you that your physical self is composed of nearly 60% water. These body fluids serve many functions, including: digestion, circulation, saliva creation, body temperature maintenance and the transport of nutrients throughout your system. These are just some of the critical services that water intake helps. Simply, your over-all good health depends on water, whether it be water from the tap filter, bottle or water-filled foods.

Calorie Control: Whether you know it or not, many times when you think you are hungry your body is actually craving from thirst. You can cut calories and start toward a more natural means to control those calories by drinking more water. Water also stimulates the metabolism, with approximately 12 ounces of the pure liquid increasing metabolism by nearly 30% for 30 minutes!

Muscle Energization: Muscle fatigue can be caused by cells

that do not maintain a balance of fluids. These cells shrivel. Water intake is an absolute necessity to quench thirsty muscles, especially before and during exercise. During exercise the water will replace the fluid loss caused by sweating.

Improved Skin Appearance: Water can keep skin toned and tight. It keeps the skin cleansed and is a natural toxin flush. The way the body works is that it naturally fills cells with water and this can reduce the appearance of wrinkles, giving your skin a naturally smooth look. Reduction of unsightly cellulite and flabby skin can also prove to be one of the benefits you can experience from sufficient water intake. You can help lock moisture in with the use of a skin moisturizer.

Kidney and Bowel Function: Drinking too little water leaves you at risk for kidney stones or kidney function that results in urine that has a foul odor and is dark in color from trapped toxins.

Your body will naturally do a remarkable job at ridding the body of toxins and cleansing your system if you drink a good amount of water. Furthermore, by keeping your body hydrated you can maintain a healthy flow through your gastrointestinal track and prevent constipation.

Healthier Hair: Cell hydration makes no exception when it comes to hydrating your hair cells as well. Your hair will begin a life that is softer and silkier if you drink your H2O.

Drinking water also reduces frizz or brittleness of the hair.

Natural Blood Thinner: You can give yourself a natural confidence boost simply by drinking more water. Faster blood flow and nourishment for your cells is the result of the blood thinning effect water has on the body. This will give you a healthier heart by reducing blood pressure and much more energy to boot. Your body will feel cleansed and in peak function performance.

Reap the Benefits! To help you increase your intake of water, drink a glass full whenever you feel dehydrated or suffer from dry mouth. Keep a bottle of water with you at all times: in the car, at the office or in your bag. This bottled water can be as simple as TAP water, provided something equivalent to a PICKLE is included with the ingestion toward PURIFICATION of the WATER itself. The amount of water you should drink will depend on your height, weight and age, but experts recommend a minimum of about 2.5 liters per day. Actually,"Pickled Water" tastes better and is more advantageous with Health Regards, due to the simultaneous intake of a "vinegar" + "veggie." Lemon or use of a Diet Lemonade Mix will also assist in increasing your water intake while helping to detox your body of impurities.

Caution: Too much PURE water can be toxic, so if you are unsure of how much you should drink you should check with your nutritionist or health care professional.

NOTE: It is typically PURIFIED water that is toxic, or can be. If you drink TAP water, there may be no limit to the amount you can consume in one day...but try not to bloat yourself. You should still check with your health care professional.

Fasting For Physical, Mental, Emotional and Spiritual Wellness

We Are So Much More than a Physical Body

It goes without saying that the magnificence which is a human being is so much more than just a physical body. Along with physical, there are emotional, mental and spiritual aspects that exist together and one should strive for wellness and harmony for total health. Fasting is one method of an effort to wellness that affects every part of our being.

While not limited to fasts that involve just water or juice, the benefits of at least an occasional fast will:

* Give the digestive system a rest

* Help you lose weight

* Allow the body to cleanse and detoxify

* Promote an increase in mental

clarity

* Heal and cleanse emotional patterns

* Increase energy level

* Enhance your spiritual connection with self by promoting an inner stillness

Fasting: The "Miracle Cure"

Many times, fasting is called the "miracle cure" because there a known and numerous physical ailments that are improved. Included in the list are arthritis, allergies, asthma, heart disease, conditions of the skin and digestive disorders of all kinds. Fasting works because it initiates the physical body's own healing mechanism and hence, ailments of almost any kind can be improved.

Fasting frees up energy so that the body can begin healing itself. When fasting, we are resting our bodies from constant intake of food. Often, eating has been thought of as a way to get energy, but actually eating requires energy. In fact, it requires a great deal of energy to digest, assimilate and metabolize the food we eat. By freeing up this energy, the energy can be diverted toward healing and recuperation.

Fasting to Lose Weight

One of the greatest benefits of fasting is the relatively rapid weight loss that can be experienced. Although professionally supervised fasts are recommended for those who suffer from serious obesity, fasting to "jump start" a new diet can change one's attitude and tastes toward more wholesome and natural foods. Fasting can also provide the insight necessary to make changes in habits and lifestyle so much more easy to accomplish.

BeNeFitS to MeNtaL aNd EMotioNaL ASpectS With FastiNg

Mental and emotional cleansing takes place when one fasts. Emotionally speaking, one can feel calmer and happier. Fasting also improves mental clarity and focus. Depressions can be lifted and obstacles, put into proper focus, can make goals appear to be more attainable. As a result of fasting, physicians have reported that their patients benefit from improved concentration, much less anxiety, better sleep and then waking with a feeling of being more refreshed.

The Spiritual Benefit of Fasting

Fasting has powerful affects on one's spiritual connection and the greater sense of kinship it can promote with one's inner being. By refraining from taking foods into the system, the physical self takes on a less dense feeling.

There begins to be a subtle separation from everyday physical reality and the worldly things it is made up of and promote the presence of things beyond the worldly - along with the power of these things.

Post-Fast Routine:

Regardless of how long or brief the fast (remember, the

LONGEST a human body can refrain from food NATURALLY and maintain naturally nourished wellness is 28 days), do not return to your "old" habits of eating. Strive to do the best you can toward eating what you 'FEEL.' This would reveal to you what your body really needs for renewed health and appropriated, more properly distributed weight. If you are unsure, DON'T EAT. Don't eat just because a clock says it is 12:00 noon or 7:30 a.m. or 5:00 p.m. Wait until you actually feel your mouth DROOL a little and try to FEEL what your

body is CRAVING for. Don't
PIG OUT. Eat slowly or until
you begin to feel full (no tummy
growl). Work toward a VEGAN
diet...and you will live
healthfully ever after.

Watch What You Eat!

Without intent intent of so yuckingly doing so, US PEOPLE have become a bunch of sh*t-heads, or otherwise known as can-a-bulls (cannibals). [Warning: Do NOT even think of that as a PRODUCT NAME - it's already called "SPAM" - so is internet Can-Spam] You say WHAT?!

 As did I upon the revelation.

 Do you realize that the PROPER and planet Respectful food

intended for the nourishment of
Human Kind is "PLANTS?"
Any meat, or meat by-product, or
dairy and dairy-product IS
SUPPOSED to make you
THROW UP! Telling us that IS
a no-no equivalent to the "Sin of
Eve in the Garden of Eden."
Fish is an in-between, to nourish
upon when major boosts of
protein are necessary [Also
Known As: 'For the Purpose of
"PIGGING OUT"' - should an
INSATIABLE CRAVING
DO-DO ARISE. So WHAT SIN
DO YOU?

Me, too.

All people should begin to graduate their eating-style to "vegan," gradually. This is not an ALARM to PANIC YOU, but just that you should REALIZE that you are "Not What You Eat," - "WHAT You EAT "CONSTITUTES" HOLY WORSHIP!" (Reference: God).

So now you say, "Oh, Sh*t!"

Well, exactly. We are all CONN-STIPULATED [Also Known as Constipated]...Who's laughing NOW Devil and "friends!"

God WILL NOT strike you dead as a result of this non-intentional "bug" type of thing in the program and coding of His Creation [Well, not up until the Judgement of Your Spirit as so determined by the Promised JUDGEMENT DAY], but when He Looked Down Upon Us [note: PAST TENSE], He said "What! What! I created a bunch of cannibals?!" But He IS sorry for the frustration, pain and sufferings us little human beans have suffered toward a "worship" of an even GREATER sin, "Vanity."

[Note: He also BLESSED those who were able to HOLD THEIR OWN and not LOSE CONTROL of themselves, regardless of faith in Conventional Religion. I.E. Not become Gluttons.]

He blames no one: For surely He has witnessed that all religions have been confused as to what to serve at their celebration tables (during rituals) and what to eat or not eat otherwise. But LIFE is a

"ritual." In fact, everything WE
DO and EVERYTHING we
consume; be it food, drink or
tobacco, should be considerate
and respectful of Him and All of
Him in His Great Glory AND
NOT to so gushingly feast for the
pleasures of our taste buds and
bellies (i.e. To BECOME
'gluttons').

So, Have a Beer! Here's to a
HAPPIER and HEALTHIER
beginning of the Promised
Eternal Physical Human Life.
The passed is OVER...THANK
GOD.

Mormon Doctrine & Covenants:

The Doctrine and Covenants

Section 89: Revelation given through Joseph Smith the Prophet, at Kirtland, Ohio, February 27, 1833. As a consequence of the early brethren using tobacco in their meetings, the Prophet was led to ponder upon the matter; consequently, he inquired of the Lord concerning it. This revelation, known as the Word of Wisdom, was the result.
1–9, The use of wine, strong

drinks, tobacco, and hot drinks is proscribed; 10–17, Herbs, fruits, flesh, and grain are ordained for the use of man and of animals; 18–21, Obedience to gospel law, including the Word of Wisdom, brings temporal and spiritual blessings.

1 A Word of Wisdom, for the benefit of the council of high priests, assembled in Kirtland, and the church, and also the saints in Zion--

2 To be sent greeting; not by

commandment or constraint, but by revelation and the word of wisdom, showing forth the order and will of God in the temporal salvation of all saints in the last days--

3 Given for a principle with promise, adapted to the capacity of the weak and the weakest of all saints, who are or can be called saints.

4 Behold, verily, thus saith the Lord unto you: In consequence of evils and designs which do and will exist in the hearts of

conspiring men in the last days, I havewarned you, and forewarn you, by giving unto you this word of wisdom by revelation--

5 That inasmuch as any man drinketh wine or strong drink among you, behold it is not good, neither meet in the sight of your Father, only in assembling yourselves together to offer up your sacraments before him.

6 And, behold, this should be wine, yea, pure wine of the grape of the vine, of your own make.

7 And, again, strong drinks are not for the belly, but for the washing of your bodies.

8 And again, tobacco is not for the body, neither for the belly, and is not good for man, but is an herb for bruises and all sick cattle, to be used with judgment and skill.

9 And again, hot drinks are not for the body or belly.

10 And again, verily I say unto you, all wholesome herbs, God hath ordained for the

constitution, nature, and use of
man--

11 Every herb in the season
thereof, and every fruit in the
season thereof; all these to be
used with prudence and
thanksgiving.

12 Yea, flesh also of beasts and
of the fowls of the air, I, the
Lord, have ordained for the use
of man with thanksgiving;
nevertheless they are to be used
sparingly;

13 And it is pleasing unto me

that they should not be used, only in times of winter, or of cold, or famine.

14 All grain is ordained for the use of man and of beasts, to be the staff of life, not only for man but for the beasts of the field, and the fowls of heaven, and all wild animals that run or creep on the earth;

15 And these hath God made for the use of man only in times of famine and excess of hunger.

16 All grain is good for the food

of man; as also the fruit of the vine; that which yieldeth fruit, whether in the ground or above the ground--

17 Nevertheless, wheat for man, and corn for the ox, and oats for the horse, and rye for the fowls and for swine, and for all beasts of the field, and barley for all useful animals, and for mild drinks, as also other grain.

18 And all saints who remember to keep and do these sayings, walking in obedience to the commandments, shall receive

health in their navel and marrow
to their bones;

19 And shall find wisdom and
great treasures of knowledge,
even hidden treasures;

20 And shall run and not be
weary, and shall walk and not
faint.

21 And I, the Lord, give unto
them a promise, that the
destroying angel shall pass by
them, as the children of Israel,
and not slay them. Amen.

Treating Constipation

You can treat constipation naturally by starting your morning with 1-2 cups of light (I use Coffeemate), sweet (I use Truvia) coffee, followed by 3 tall glasses of filtered water.

If you find you have still not moved your bowels by early to mid-afternoon, repeat the coffee treatment.

For severe cases, I use children's laxative suppositories for the gentlest relief.

THe MagicaL WiNdoWS oF tHe MiNd

Popular Belief:

Contrary to the popular belief
that the eyes serve as the
windows to the Soul, in fact the
eyes are the windows to a Mind
that have made a Soul
Connection. When vision
becomes impaired, whether slight
mal-focusing to acute blindness,
it indicates that the mind needs to
heal. The process of the mind
healing is a very delicate task

that only God can undertake. The best bet that I have found is to wear spectacles that will slowly and gradually refocus the injured eyes as they begin readjusting themselves to the acceptance of light, such as sunlight.

An Amazing Discovery - A Personal Experience
Throughout my life, I have had difficulty with clear vision, usually nearsightedness, as a result of a severe case of German Measles. I tried avoiding the use of eyeglasses, thinking they

would make me unattractive
during my formative years, until I
entered the ranks of the duly
employed. At that point, I
invested in contact lenses and
wore them every day. My vision
was temporarily improved, but
the lenses did not serve as any
corrective measure to my poor,
injured eyes.

One day, a calamity of
circumstances landed me in a
Forensic Hospital. One of the
medical exams that they felt
necessary was an examination of
the eyes. I sat in the examination

chair and the doctor kept adjusting the prospective lenses while I made the effort to read the standard eye chart, top to bottom. When a particular adjustment was made, I proceeded to read the ENTIRE eye chart, including the achievement of reading the very, very bottom line (intrinsic focus required).

This ability was a first in my entire lifetime. Needless to say, I was very excited. When the associated, single focal spectacles were made and delivered to me, I continually practiced looking and focusing on everything in sight. I was truly amazed at the things I saw.

Discernation:

Many years have passed since the days when my perfect vision glasses were the popular style and the only glasses I needed to wear. Eye exams led to bi-focals, tri-focals and progressives. My vision started to once again decline. I could feel the strain and the ineptness in proper focusing. These inept products of popular style were hurting, not helping, my ability to see.

Aside from learning that near-sightedness is a result of physical (body) "trauma" and not able to see far is indicative of a traumatized mind that needs to heal, I prefer 2 separate, single lens glasses - as prescribed toward improvement of both. With continued use of my perfect vision glasses, it was found necessary that I needed a lens combination for distance (such as for proper concentration while driving) and another for reading (such as for use of a computer).

My perfect vision glasses were PERFECT. This would mean a style round and wide enough to heal and protect direct line vision and full sphere peripherals. To each his own. But I still believe there is nothing wrong with being a little old-fashioned, even if a little goofy looking in style. One must have a sense of humor about life. For, surely, life is more important than mere aesthetics.

Note: To this day I possess my pair of MAGIC single focus all around perfect vision glasses. They will ALWAYS work - because I SAW 100% with a single lens. The difficulty is maintaining concentration when needed urgently, such as for working on my computer or driving. These are times when concentration absolute could be absolutely critical. The reason is that FROM THERE (perfect vision glasses), it's only BETTER AND BETTER as life and body evolve inward toward the future and toward outward beauty: Inward serenity and outward beauty reflected ALL from the spirit of God felt within.

PSaLM 23:
KiNg JaMeS VerSioN (KJV)

The Lord is my shepherd; I shall not want.

He maketh me to lie down in green pastures: he leadeth me beside the still waters.

He restoreth my soul: he leadeth me in the paths of righteousness for his name's sake.

Yea, though I walk through the

valley of the shadow of death, I will fear no evil: for thou art with me; thy rod and thy staff they comfort me.

Thou preparest a table before me in the presence of mine enemies: thou anointest my head with oil; my cup runneth over.

Surely goodness and mercy shall follow me all the days of my life: and I will dwell in the house of the Lord for ever.

NoW it MuSt be DiScuSSed: PHySiCaL ScieNce (PHySiciaNS)

The Physical Science of Human Beings is a difficult subject to approach, mainly due to personal fears of physical intrusion and/or possible desecration of some delicate aspect to mine own human body. But these practitioners are a necessary "evil," if you may, in order for a diverse and volatile genetics of beings to evolve to maturity - and possibly beyond.

There is a natural order to all

things and the sciences are no exception. Highest order is Omni Science, relative to God. Second is the Physical Science of Human Beings, which practitioners are known as Physicians or Doctors and including, Dentists (or any variation thereof).

Proper practitioners are well aware of their authorities and responsibilities and strive to protect the personal privacy of their entrusted patients. They do not spew lies, but rather offer intelligent and caring advice and recommendations, typically subsequent to exam and sometimes "tests." Proper practitioners do not PLAY GOD, for they are aware that their knowledge, however current, is still only a HISTORY of evolutionary events. It is always the patient's RIGIIT to REFUSE a doctor's opinion, REFUSE "tests," and/or seek opinion elsewhere.

To me, doctor's have played a role of TRUSTED GUIDANCE councellors, when I feared an ailment of body was beyond "doing without" more

knowledgeable care. Although, I
admit, I am guilty of not
adhering to a "routine" "question
and answer" periods with general
practitioners. I do not even like
"giving" blood, which is
probably the most painless and
basic "test" a practitioner needs.
I believe adamantly in God, and
have always believed the God
Himself was the only doctor I
would ever need. However, I
have learned that "things happen"
that are beyond a human's control
and God cannot manifest hands
small enough to tend to intricate
details.

There is one specific type of doctor I would rather die than to visit routinely and that is anyone who claims to be a "female" or "woman" doctor (Gynochologists). Like my belief that God is the general Doctor of my Body, I feel a Husband should be the Doctor of my womanly parts. I feel regular intrusion into the most delicate and misunderstood area of human being (womanly parts) is not only desecration, but worse than the sin of something as innocent as masterbation. Of course, intrusion or desecration would be a husband's decision to make, should a LOVING husband have cause for concern. But in general I would have to say this is one aspect of medicine that should be thought long and hard about - comparative to possibly a worst of all sin - before tampering or toying with God's "baby making machine," especially an unmarried woman who has not advice of a loving husband.

The last, and probably the most critical, aspect of the Science of Human Being Health is that which pertains to the Human Mind. Supplementary to my book, "The Spirit Cries," it has been discerned that there are only three "states" of "mind" in the present tense. The first is "Serenity." Serenity is marked by an extreme "peace of mind" that is achieved when a human's "body, spirit and soul" have found an acute balance. This is a state of "good health." The final two are difficult to diagnose in difference: A State of "Trauma" and a State of being "Mentally Ill." "Trauma" is a state of mind experience when the mind is

injured. "Mental Illness" is a
state of degeneration. Where a
mind can heal from Trauma (for
example, Post Traumatic Stress
Syndrome"), there is no cure for
"Mental Illness." These 3 states
are the 3 DIMENSIONS of a
living being.

There are 5 dimensions. The
fourth dimension is commonly
referred to as the CURRENCY
of DEATH. Depending upon
what state of mind an individual
achieves in present tense, the
fourth dimension can also be
predicate of a physical and

spiritual "re-birth," which state is brief. It is usually followed surely and quickly by an entry into the 5th dimension...the state where eternal, physical human life is achieved. "Mentally Ill" individuals will never achieve the spiritual state of the 4th dimension that permits "re-birth," and will therefore be "stuck" at the 4th dimensionary death. This is because their minds CANNOT heal, and de-evolve as they de-generate FREQUENCY.

Dentistry would be the highest of all of the human being doctor sciences, for without teeth, or prospect thereof, there WOULD BE no connection between body, mind and spirit - nor heart. What will happen, will happen - but teeth should be kept in original form unless pain becomes unbearable. Fillings would be first, with a last resort of pulling of the teeth. Final resort would be dentures, but one must be aware that with dentures there is no psychoanalytics, as typically the roof of the mouth is cut off from the powers of the mind that exist in the brain. For God Sake, never cap or alter your two front teeth for the simple reason of aesthetics. As they represent the connection of the heart and doing so can suffocate one to death. The two front teeth must BREATHE or BREATH is cut off.

It's a New Life: How to Begin

You will probably want to start your new life with a little "feel good" shopping spree at your local Walmart - or shop online if you don't want to roam through the hugeness of the store or don't have transportation. Keep in mind that I am a woman. Men, typically, can do what is comfortable and comes naturally.

1) New Undergarments:

   Under Panties: I buy Hanes cotton briefs and use "U" by

Kotex (long, ultra thin, wrapped pads) as a regular panty liner. I do not waste water by doing laundry often, but the underwear is inexpensive enough to buy 30 pair (wearing a pair for approximately 1 week, changing pad as necessary). My under panties are white, which color attracts impurities from a woman's private parts. A daily natural cleaning takes place as impurities are naturally distracted away.

Bras: I wear Fruit of the Loom sports bra, front closure, for typically every day. Color is basically unimportant for sport. But there are times when I want a little more of a "Smart & Sexy" look, for which I treated myself to "Smart & Sexy" everyday romantics, color white, which will also attract impurities from delicate mammaries, since a little "squeezing" is involved.

2) Everyday "Home Hang" Casual Clothing:

I typically wear oversized men's cotton t-shirts, or plus-sized women's tee's. My bust

size is 36D, but my t-shirt size is
2X. I wear 3X white, men's tee's
to bed (commonly keeping my
sport bra on, to delay breast
sagging and rejuvenate support).
I still typically purchase oversized shirts, even for "office" or
"outings." But this time I will
buy women's shirts, in colourful
colors and designs, size 2X.

At "home," during most
weather, I wear comfortable
"stretch" jeans. For "office" or
"outings" (when I am not just
running to the store or places
where jeans may be prohibited), I

wear, comfortable and oversized if necessary, elastic waist slacks. Danskin has nice slacks, which may be something new at this writing, called "Danskin Now, Dri-More Core."

Generally, I don't like to put pressure on my belly, as a woman is prone, even when aging, to "puffy," womanly ways.

For summer, or days when long jeans are just "too" hot, I wear men's boxers. They come in a variety of colors and prints and the little slit in front is cool, too ("puff up," always remember). Hanes, again, is affordable - but a boxer is a boxer. Even all white is smart and clean.

Regardless of "home" or "outing," on my feet I wear ankle high, typically white socks. Hanes has a "Comfortable Collection - Cool & Dry - Ankle." But usually, any Hanes anklet is sufficient. Feet are very important. "Cool & Dry" is really VERY COOL!

For shoes, my favorite and most comfortable are, believe it or not, Keds "sneaker like," lace up shoes. They are not as sloppy as sneakers and I can wear them most everywhere, including "office." I absolutely avoid "high heels." Another, more "dressy" favorite shoe is the old-fashioned "saddle shoe." You may have to search under "costumes" for a pair, but they are truly the BEST shoes for your feet. They must be broken in, but once they are fit to your feet, you will find no other shoe with such good support that is a "dressy" look. I had to buy mine from the costume shoppe, so the inner souls are not the best. Simple. I used Dr. Scholl's "aqua" (gelly water) liners. Now my "saddles" are great!

3) Grooming & Daily or Every Other Day Routine:

Basic "Bathroom" Supplies -

*Colgate gel toothpaste;
*A Medium Bristle toothbrush;
*A thin, round, hair brush;
*White Face cloths;
*Hydrogen Peroxide;

*"Pretty Feet" Exfoliant Rough Skin Remover by B.F. Ascher & Co.;
*Johnson's Baby Lotion;
*Men's Speed Stick (regular) Deodorant by Mennen;
*"Irish Spring" soap;
*Suave "Ocean Breeze" Shampoo;
*Stridex Daily Care Alcohol-Free Sensitive with Aloe Pads;
*Anti-Bacterial hand soft soap;
*Lady Shick disposable razors.

Start Your New Life:

Start your new life with an "as hot as you can comfortably stand" shower. Wear "hospital style" traction slipper socks on your feet. You will need soap and shampoo. That's it. First, wash your hair and rinse thoroughly. Then soap down your body, making sure you soap up your belly button and thoroughly soap your private area, without any penetration. Then, your legs and behind. Soap up your hands, then, and wash your face, ears and neck.

Don't go INTO your ear, just the outer ear. Careful not to get water in your ear, this could cause infection. I use earplugs.

The "quick" shower should not take more than 10-15 minutes. Don't waste water on unnecessary luxury - and don't waste money on shower luxury, either. The purpose is cleaning - not worshiping of your body.

Once rinsed off thoroughly, step our of the shower and remove your slipper socks. Towel dry your hair and then, using the same towel, quickly and gently dry the drip off your body. After shower, step into your under panties, lined, a fresh pair and throw on one of your nighttime super sized men's tee's. Proceed to brush out your hair. DON'T USE A HAIR DRYER. Let locks dry naturally. When to a point of "damp," you can "set" your hair, or trim your bangs, if you have them. I set my hair making braids, for wave or Swahili cool-look. All I use are some "scunci" effortless beauty elastics, with no metal parts and for no damage.

After you are dry, if you are at the beginning or afternoon of your day, apply deoderant and dress. If not, your ready for a clean nite's sleep.

I typically conserve water, so I only shower AT MOST once a week. But I have gone longer, using "pretty feet," hydrogen peroxide on a face cloth for my belly, legs and arms (and sometimes face), and Stridex pads on my face. Do not use hydrogen peroxide on your mammaries or private parts. The stomach area is as far as I go.

But you will feel fresh and clean and realize you don't need a shower - to wash away 'DEAD SKIN CELLS' yet. Follow up on your feet, legs, arms and wherever with baby lotion.

In the morning I brush my teeth AND TONGUE, making sure to brush my gums. I wear dentures. I wash/brush them with liquid hand soap.

From time to time, I may notice some facial hair. I use my Lady Shick, including for my eyebrows. No point plucking.

Besides, it's painful and I am not a masochist. Other unwanted hair (legs/armpits), I would also use my Lady Shick.

For finger nails, I keep mine short and clean dirt from under with free fingers, sometimes under water using a little hand soap. Again, I am not such a masochist that I would scrape my sensitive undernails with sharp metals.

I also watch my toenail. Keeping them trim so that they are comfortable in my shoes.